Competitive Foods and Beverages in U.S. Schools

A State Policy Analysis

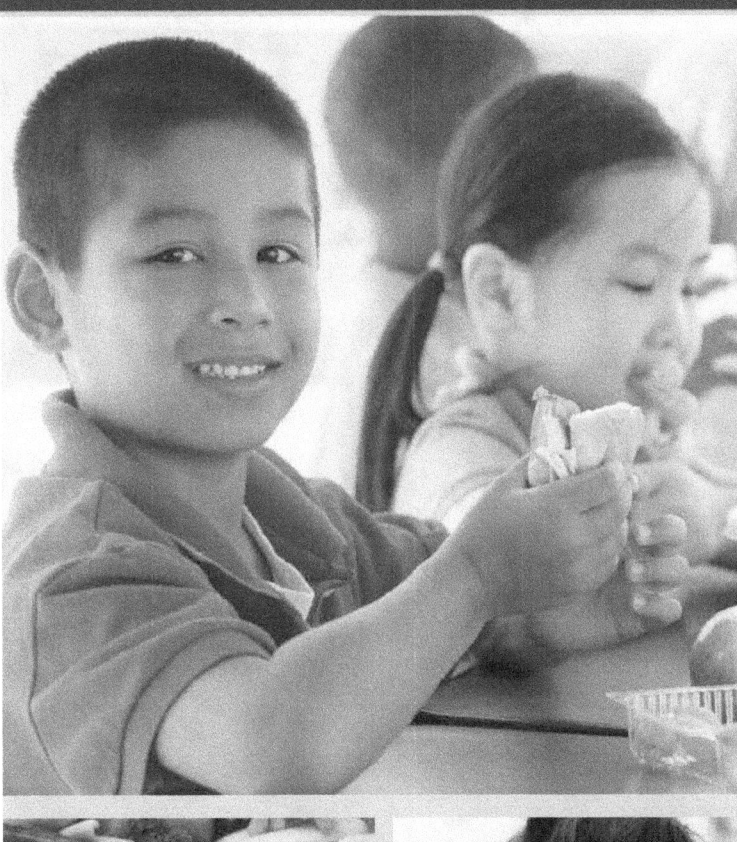

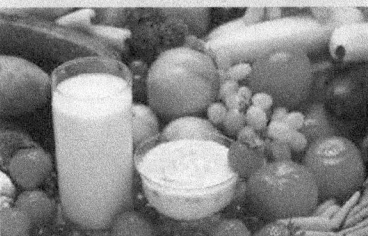

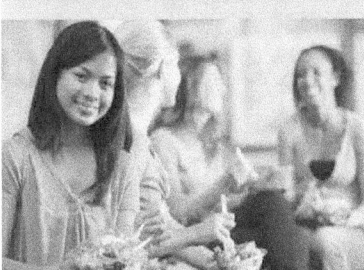

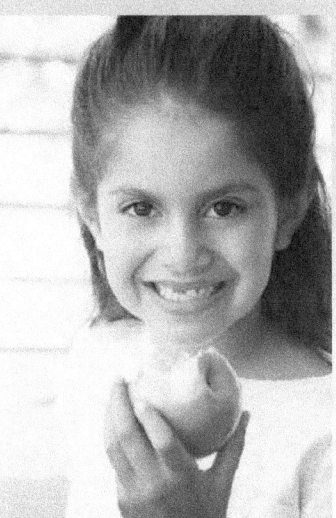

National Center for Chronic Disease Prevention and Health Promotion

Division of Population Health

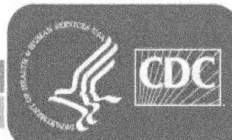

For more information, please contact
Division of Population Health
National Center for Chronic Disease Prevention and Health Promotion
Centers for Disease Control and Prevention
1600 Clifton Road, NE, Mailstop A-11; TTY: 1-888-232-6348
Phone: 1-800-CDC-INFO (232-4636)
Web site: www.cdc.gov/healthyyouth

Suggested Citation

Centers for Disease Control and Prevention. *Competitive Foods and Beverages in U.S. Schools: A State Policy Analysis*. Atlanta: U.S. Department of Health and Human Services; 2012.

Competitive Foods and Beverages in U.S. Schools

A State Policy Analysis

Contents

Introduction

Since 1980, the prevalence of obesity among U.S. children and adolescents has tripled, and today 19.6% of children aged 6–11 years and 18.1% of adolescents aged 12–19 years are categorized as obese.[1] Because youth spend a significant amount of their day in school, it is an ideal venue to promote obesity prevention efforts. A growing body of research has found that the school food environment is associated with youth dietary behaviors and obesity.[2-6]

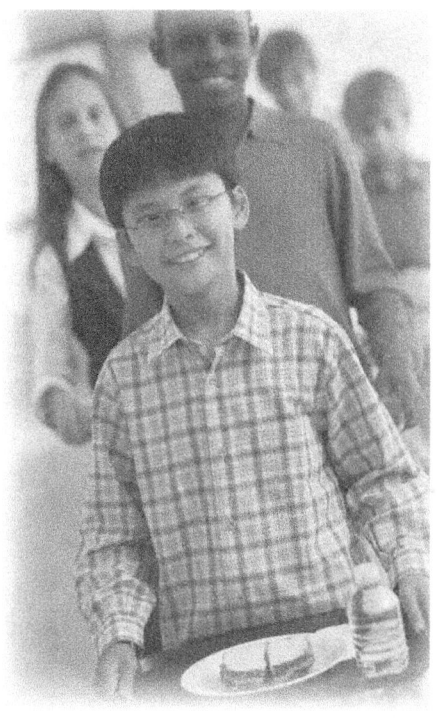

Schools can play a critical role by establishing a safe and supportive environment with policies and practices that sustain healthy behaviors. In addition, schools provide opportunities for youth to learn about and practice healthy eating and physical activity.

U.S. students are exposed to a broad range of foods and beverages through reimbursable school meals, à la carte lines, vending machines, school stores, classroom parties, fundraisers, and other school events. Nutrition standards for federally reimbursable school meals are regulated by the U.S. Department of Agriculture's National School Lunch Program and School Breakfast Program.[7,8] Current federal regulations for competitive foods, which are those foods sold or available in schools outside of federally reimbursable school meals programs, prohibit the sale of foods of minimal nutritional value (FMNV) (e.g., chewing gum, carbonated soft drinks, certain candies) during meal periods in the food service area, where reimbursable school meals are sold or eaten.[7,8] However, no federal regulations exist for other competitive foods that are also high in calories, fat, sodium, and sugar, but which are not specifically identified as FMNV.

In December 2010, Congress enacted the Healthy, Hunger-Free Kids Act of 2010, which requires the development of federal nutrition standards for all competitive foods sold in schools. (For more information, see www.gpo.gov/fdsys/pkg/BILLS-111s3307enr/pdf/BILLS-111s3307enr.pdf.)

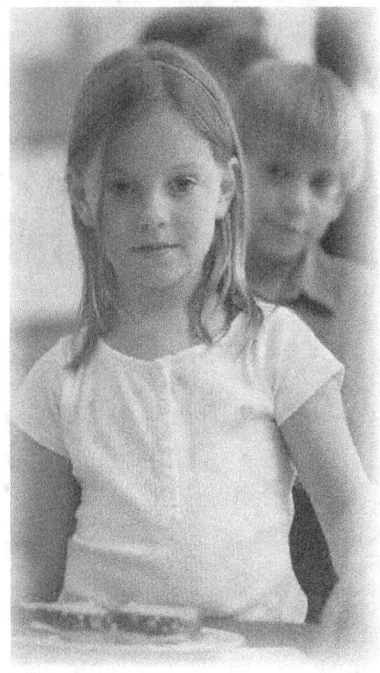

Competitive foods and beverages are widely available in schools.[4,9] State and local education agencies have the ability to set rules for competitive foods (including FMNV) that are more stringent than federal regulations. For example, states can prohibit the sale of FMNV on the entire school campus for the entire school day, or they can set policies regulating the nutritional content of all competitive foods and beverages in schools.

The Healthy, Hunger-Free Kids Act of 2010 also requires local educational agencies to include nutrition guidelines for competitive foods in schools as part of their local wellness policies. However, because federal officials have not had the authority to create required standards for the content of these guidelines, local policies for competitive foods vary widely in strength and comprehensiveness.[10]

Purpose

CDC analyzed requirements included in state laws, regulations, and policies related to the availability and nutritional content of competitive foods in schools on the basis of how closely they align with the recommendations in the Institute of Medicine's (IOM's) *Nutrition Standards for Foods in Schools: Leading the Way Toward Healthier Youth* (IOM Standards).[11] The IOM Standards for competitive foods and beverages in schools are not required by any federal mandate, but they serve as the gold standard recommendations for the availability, sale, and content of competitive foods in schools.

The IOM Standards report concluded that

- Federally reimbursable school meals programs should be the main source of nutrition in schools.

- Opportunities for competitive foods should be limited.

- If competitive foods are available, they should consist primarily of fruits, vegetables, whole grains, and nonfat or low-fat milk and milk products.

Institute of Medicine Nutrition Standards for Foods in Schools

Standards for Nutritive Food Components

1. Snacks, foods, and beverages meet dietary fat criteria per portion as packaged: no more than 35% of total calories from fat, less than 10% of total calories from saturated fat, and zero trans fat.

2. Snacks, foods, and beverages provide no more than 35% of calories from total sugars per portion as packaged. Exceptions to the standard are

    a. 100% fruits and fruit juices in all forms without added sugars.

    b. 100% vegetables and vegetable juices without added sugars.

    c. Unflavored nonfat and low-fat milk and yogurt. Flavored nonfat and low-fat milk can contain no more than 22 grams of total sugars per 8-ounce portion, and flavored nonfat and low-fat yogurt can contain no more than 30 grams of total sugars per 8-ounce serving.

3. Snack items are 200 calories or less per portion as packaged, and à la carte entrée items do not exceed calorie limits on comparable National School Lunch Program (NSLP) items.

4. Snack items meet a sodium content limit of 200 mg or less per portion as packaged or 480 mg or less per entrée portion as served à la carte.

Standards for Nonnutritive Food Components

5. Beverages containing nonnutritive sweeteners are only allowed in high schools after the end of the school day.

6. Foods and beverages are caffeine-free, with the exception of trace amounts of naturally occurring caffeine-related substances.

Standards for the School Day

7. Foods and beverages offered during the school day are limited to those in Tier 1.

8. Plain, potable water is available throughout the school day at no cost to students.

9. Sport drinks are not available in the school setting except when provided by the school for student athletes participating in sport programs involving vigorous activity of more than 1 hour's duration.

10. Foods and beverages are not used as rewards or discipline for academic performance or behavior.

11. Minimize marketing of Tier 2 snacks, foods, and beverages in the high school setting by locating Tier 2 food and beverage distribution in low student traffic areas and ensuring that the exteriors of vending machines do not depict commercial products or logos or suggest that consumption of vended items conveys health or social benefit.

Standards for the After-School Setting

12. Tier 1 snack items are allowed after school for student activities for elementary and middle schools. Tier 1 and 2 snacks are allowed after school for high school.

13. For on-campus fundraising activities during the school day, Tier 1 foods and beverages are allowed for elementary, middle, and high schools. Tier 2 foods and beverages are allowed for high schools after school. For evening and community activities that include adults, Tier 1 and 2 foods and beverages are encouraged.

Definitions

Tier 1 foods and beverages for all students. **Tier 1 foods** are fruits, vegetables, whole grains, and related combination products, and nonfat and low-fat dairy products that are limited to ≤200 calories per portion as packaged and ≤35% of total calories from fat, <10% of total calories from saturated fats, zero trans fat (≤0.5 g per serving), ≤35% of calories from total sugars, and ≤200 mg sodium. À la carte entrée items meet fat and sugar limits as listed above.

Tier 1 beverages are water without flavoring, additives, or carbonation; low-fat and nonfat milk in 8-oz portions, including lactose-free and soy beverages and flavored milk with no more than 22 g of total sugars per 8-oz portion; 100% fruit juice in 4-oz portions as packaged for elementary/middle school and 8-oz portions for high school; and caffeine-free, with the exception of trace amounts of naturally occurring caffeine substances.

Tier 2 foods and beverages are any foods or beverages for high school students after school. Tier 2 snack foods are those that do not exceed 200 calories per portion as packaged and ≤35% of total calories from fat, <10% of total calories from saturated fats, zero trans fat (≤0.5 g per serving), ≤35% calories from total sugars, and a sodium content of ≤200 mg per portion as packaged. Tier 2 beverages are noncaffeinated, nonfortified beverages with <5 calories per portion as packaged, with or without nonnutritive sweeteners, carbonation, or flavoring.

Methods

Several sources were used to identify state laws, regulations, and policies enacted prior to October 1, 2010, that govern the availability of competitive foods and beverages in schools. These sources included the official state government Web sites for all 50 states, the National Association of State Boards of Education's Health Policies database, and the National Conference of State Legislatures' Childhood Obesity database. Thirty-nine states have such laws, regulations, or policies, and copies of relevant state policy documents were obtained, including codified laws, state board of education policies, memos, and resolutions for analysis. Eleven states did not have any laws, regulations, or policies related to competitive foods in schools. For this report, the word *policy* is used as an umbrella term encompassing a state law, regulation, or state board of education policy.

To guide the analysis, CDC researchers developed and piloted a codebook based on the IOM Standards. Each of the 13 IOM Standards was divided into variables to reflect the complexity of the standard. For example, IOM Standard 1 is divided into 3 variables, and IOM Standard 7 is divided into 11 variables. This process weighted Standard 7 more heavily than the others because it encompasses the majority of standards related to the nutritional quality of competitive foods. The process resulted in 33 variables; 28 were applicable for elementary and middle schools, and 32 were applicable for high schools (Appendix A).

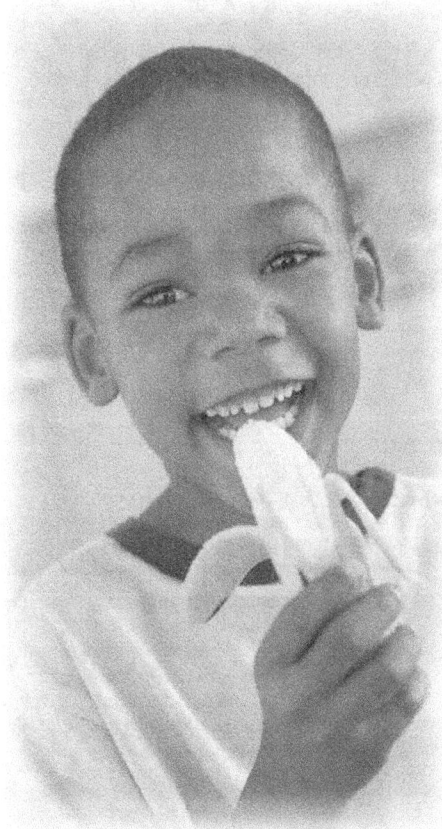

Each of the variables was defined and coded based on the following general rating system, similar to the coding methodology used elsewhere:[10]

0 = Variable not mentioned in state policy or is not required.

1 = Variable is mentioned in the state policy, but only partially meets the variable definition or does not apply to entire school campus or entire school day, or only a certain percentage of foods or beverages are required to meet the variable definition.

2 = Variable is mentioned and fully meets or exceeds the variable definition and applies to the entire school campus and the entire school day, or competitive foods are banned.

For example, when coding a policy for the calories variable that snack items must contain 200 calories or less per portion as packaged, the policy would receive a "1" rating if it mentions lowering calories for snacks but does not include a specific calorie level or only sets portion size limits for certain snack foods. For this same variable, a state policy would receive a "2" rating if it requires all snacks available on the school campus to be limited to 200 calories or less per portion as packaged.

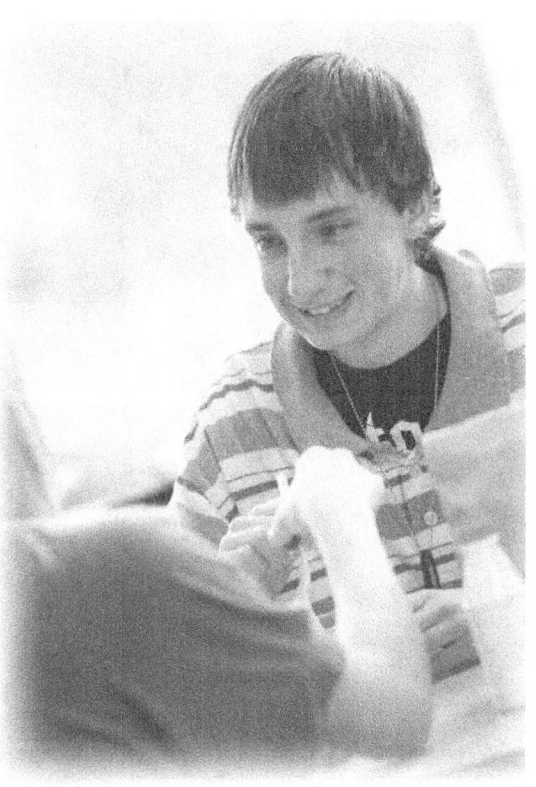

CDC researchers independently reviewed and coded the state policy documents for the 33 variables separately for each grade level—elementary, middle, and high school (if applicable). Differences in coding were resolved through discussion and consensus between the CDC researchers or by another subject matter expert.

State policies were analyzed to determine how closely they align with IOM Standards. Overall alignment scores were determined for each state policy, across all school levels combined, and at each of the three different school levels separately. Alignment scores were calculated by adding the sum of scores for each applicable variable, dividing by the maximum possible score (i.e., 176 across all school levels, 56 at the elementary and middle school levels, and 64 at the high school level), and multiplying by 100 for ease of interpretation.

A similar analysis looked only at the variables derived from the first 9 IOM Standards because they specifically address the nutrient content of foods and beverages available during the school day. The maximum alignment scores for the nutrient standards only analysis were calculated by adding the sum of scores for each applicable variable, dividing by the maximum possible score, (i.e., 140 across all school levels, 46 at the elementary and middle school levels, and 48 at the high school level) and multiplying by 100 for ease of interpretation.

State policy alignment scores were then categorized into quartiles (see below). For both analyses, the higher the score and corresponding quartile, the greater the alignment with IOM Standards.

Quartile 1   0–25.0
Quartile 2   25.1–50.0
Quartile 3   50.1–75.0
Quartile 4   75.1–100.0

In addition, each state policy's alignment score is accompanied by the number of IOM Standards that are met in the policy, either fully or partially—identified as the scope of the state policy. To fully meet an IOM Standard, a state policy had to score a "2" (the maximum score) for all applicable variables at each school level. To partially meet an IOM Standard, a state policy had to score a "1" on any of the applicable variables at any grade level. The more IOM Standards that were fully or partially met, the greater the scope of the state policy.

Key Findings

Description of State Policies

- As of October 1, 2010, 78% of the nation (39 states) had enacted state policies for competitive foods in schools. Specifically,

  » 27 states had policies that require schools to implement nutrition standards for competitive foods and beverages. In Connecticut, standards for beverages are required, but competitive food standards are voluntary.

  » 2 states (Massachusetts and Virginia) had recently enacted legislation to develop state nutrition requirements for competitive foods in schools, but no standards existed as of October 1, 2010.

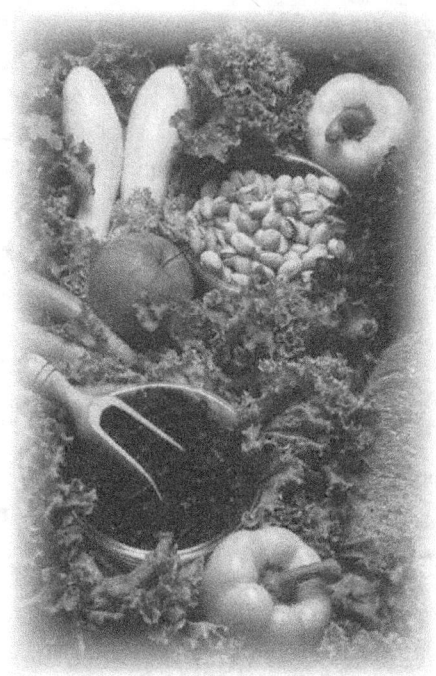

  » 4 states (Michigan, Pennsylvania, Utah, and Vermont) had policies that recommend but do not require schools to implement nutrition standards for competitive foods.

  » 6 states (Delaware, Georgia, Maine, Maryland, New York, and Oklahoma) had policies that only restrict the time and place of the sale of FMNV at certain school levels that go beyond current federal regulations for FMNV.

- 23 states had policies that were enacted before 2007, when the IOM Standards report was released.

- 33 states had policies that include standards for each of the 3 school levels (elementary, middle, and high school).

- 4 states (Arizona, Illinois, Oklahoma, and Tennessee) had policies that apply only to the elementary and middle school levels.

- 2 states (Georgia and South Carolina) had policies that apply only to elementary schools.

- 2 states (Indiana and North Carolina) banned vending machines in elementary schools.

- 2 states (Arkansas and Florida) banned all competitive foods and beverages in elementary schools throughout the entire school day and campus.

- 2 states (Colorado and Connecticut) had policies for beverages only.

Overall Alignment Scores

No state policy fully met all of the IOM Standards (all 33 variables assessed). Therefore, no state policy had alignment scores in the 4th quartile (Figure 1). The majority of state policies had alignment scores in the 1st or 2nd quartile.

- 2 states (Hawaii and West Virginia) had alignment scores in the 3rd quartile.

- 18 state policies had alignment scores in the 2nd quartile.

- 19 state policies had alignment scores in the 1st quartile.

Table 1 (see page 10) shows each state's overall alignment score for all schools levels combined and for each school level separately.

Figure 1. Alignment of State Policies for Competitive Foods and Beverages in Schools with IOM Standards, All IOM Standards (N = 39 States)

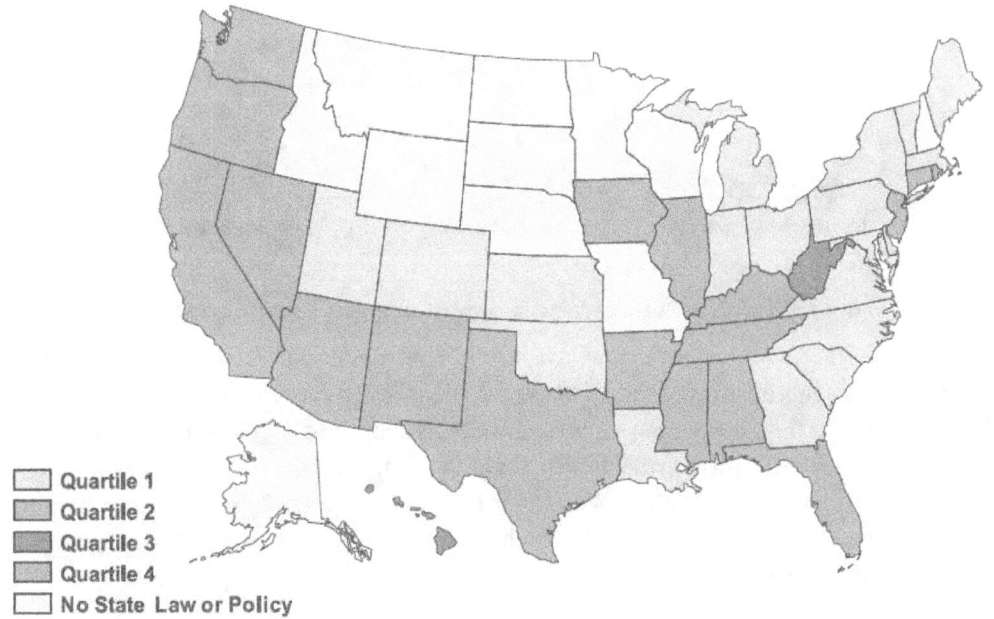

Quartile 1
Quartile 2
Quartile 3
Quartile 4
No State Law or Policy

Overall Alignment Scores by School Level

In most states, policies for competitive foods in middle and high schools had lower alignment scores than those for elementary schools (Table 1 and Figure 2). Although most state policies for elementary schools required 100% of foods and beverages to meet state standards, some state policies for middle and high schools only required a certain percentage (e.g., 50%) of foods or beverages to meet state standards, resulting in a lower alignment score.

As Figure 2 illustrates, 4 states (Hawaii, Iowa, Mississippi, and West Virginia) had policies for elementary schools in the 3rd quartile, compared with only 2 states (Hawaii and West Virginia) in the 3rd quartile for middle and high school levels. Arkansas and Florida were the only states with policies for elementary schools in the 4th quartile. Both of these states banned all competitive foods and beverages in elementary schools.

Figure 2. Number and Alignment Score of State Policies for Competitive Foods in Each Quartile, All IOM Standards, by School Level (N = 39 States)

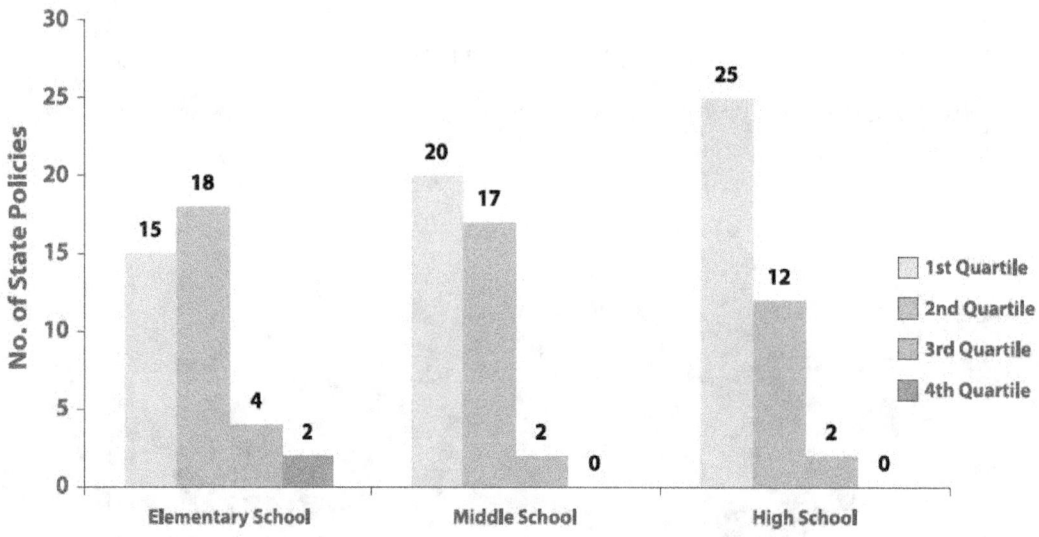

Alignment Scores of Food and Beverage Nutrient Standards by School Level

Table 1 provides the alignment score for each state in meeting the 24 variables that make up the nutrient standards subset (IOM Standards 1–9) for all school levels combined and separately for each school level. In this subset analysis, all school levels combined, 1 state policy (Hawaii) had an alignment score in the 4th quartile. Five states (Alabama, Arkansas, Iowa, Mississippi, and West Virginia) had policies with alignment scores in the 3rd quartile, 20 states had policies with alignment scores in the 2nd quartile, and 14 states had policies with alignment scores in the 1st quartile, indicating the least alignment with IOM Standards.

Figure 3 shows the number of state policies in each quartile for this subset of standards by school level. State policy provisions for food and beverage nutrient standards were more aligned with IOM Standards at the elementary school level than middle and high school levels. Seven states had alignment scores for elementary school in the 3rd quartile, compared with 5 states for middle school, and 2 states for high school. Arkansas, Florida, and Hawaii's alignment scores for elementary school were in the 4th quartile, indicating the greatest alignment with IOM Standards. For this subset analysis, Hawaii was the only state whose policy was in the 4th quartile (greatest alignment with IOM Standards) for each grade level.

Figure 3. Number and Alignment Score of State Policies for Competitive Foods in Schools in Each Quartile, by School Level, Nutrient Standards Only (Standards 1–9), (N = 39 States)

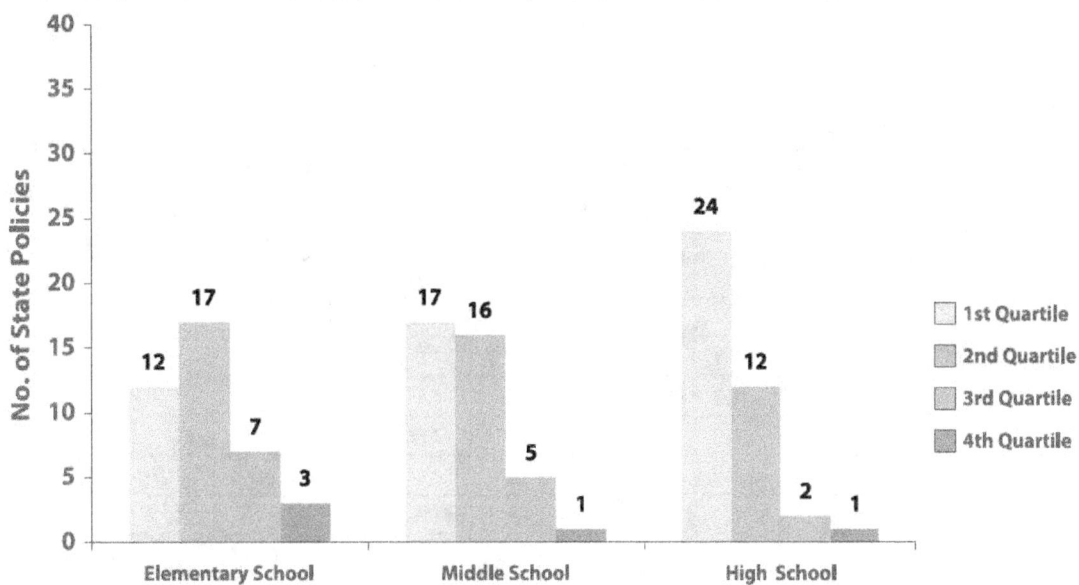

Scope of State Policies

The scope of each state's policies is a reflection of policy content (i.e., how many IOM Standards, fully or partially met, are included in a policy). The larger the number of IOM Standards that are fully or partially met, the greater the scope of the state policy. Table 1 provides details about the scope of each state policy. In summary,

- The scope of state policies ranged from 0–12 out of 13 IOM Standards.

- Table 1 shows that states can have lower alignment scores with a broad scope. For example, Tennessee's overall alignment score is 31.1 (out of 100, 2nd quartile), but its policy addresses 11 out of the 13 IOM Standards (a broad scope).

- The 5 states with the broadest scope were West Virginia (12 standards), Hawaii (11 standards), Tennessee (10 standards), Arkansas (10 standards), Iowa (9 standards), Arizona (9 standards), and Alabama (9 standards).

- The 2 states with the greatest alignment with IOM Standards (all IOM Standards) also had a broad scope: West Virginia (12 standards) and Hawaii (11 standards).

- Of the states with lower alignment scores (i.e. in the 1st quartile [N = 19]), 14 states partially met 1–8 of the 13 IOM Standards. The remaining 5 states did not meet or partially meet any IOM Standards because the standards in the state policies are not required or had not been developed at the time of analysis.

Table 1. Alignment Score by School Level and Scope of State Policies for Competitive Foods and Beverages in U.S. Schools

State	Alignment Scores of State Policies with IOM Standards								Scope of State Policies		
	Overall Score[a] (out of 100)				Nutrient Standards Only Score[b] (out of 100)						
	All School Levels	E	M	H	All School Levels	E	M	H	No. of IOM Standards Fully Met (out of 13)	No. of IOM Standards Partially Met (out of 13)	Total Scope
Alabama	43.2	48.2	46.4	35.9	51.4	56.5	54 3	43.8	0	9	9
Alaska[c]											
Arizona	27.3	44.6	41.1	0	32.9	52.2	47.8	0	0	9	9
Arkansas	46.6	85.7	30.4	26.6	51.4	95.7	30.4	29.2	1	9	10
California	41.5	48.2	39 3	37.5	47.1	54.3	43 5	43.8	1	7	8
Colorado	23.3	26.8	26.8	17.2	24 3	28.3	28 3	16.7	0	6	6
Connecticut[d]	29.5	30.4	30.4	28.1	35.0	34.8	34.8	35.4	1	7	8
Delaware[e]	1.7	1.8	1.8	1.6	2.1	2 2	2.2	2.1	0	1	1
Florida	27.3	78.6	3.6	3.1	34 3	95.7	4.3	4.2	0	8	8
Georgia[e]	1.1	3.6	0	0	1.4	4 3	0	0	0	1	1
Hawaii	70.5	71.4	71.4	68.8	76.4	76.1	76.1	77.1	5	6	11
Idaho[c]											
Illinois	26.1	41.1	41.1	0	31.4	47.8	47.8	0	0	6	6
Indiana	21.6	25.0	21.4	18.8	25.0	28.3	23.9	22.9	0	8	8
Iowa	47.7	55.4	46.4	42.2	57.9	65.2	54 3	54.2	3	6	9
Kansas	21.0	25.0	25.0	14.1	24 3	28.3	28 3	16.7	0	6	6
Kentucky	30.7	32.1	32.1	28.1	36.4	37.0	37.0	35.4	1	6	7
Louisiana	22.7	32.1	19.6	17.2	28.6	39.1	23.9	22.9	0	6	6
Maine[e]	8.0	7.1	7.1	9.4	8.6	8.7	8.7	8.3	0	1	1
Maryland[e]	3.4	3.6	3.6	3.1	4.3	4 3	4.3	4.2	0	4	4
Massachusetts[f]	8.5	8.9	8.9	7.8	10.7	10.9	10.9	10.4	0	2	2
Michigan[d]	0	0	0	0	0	0	0	0	0	0	0
Minnesota[c]											
Mississippi	46.6	51.8	48 2	40.6	53.6	58.7	54 3	47.9	0	7	7
Missouri[c]											
Montana[c]											
Nebraska[c]											
Nevada	30.1	33.9	30.4	26.6	33.6	37.0	32.6	31.3	0	8	8
New Hampshire[c]											
New Jersey	25.6	30.4	25.0	21.9	27.9	32.6	26.1	25.0	0	6	6
New Mexico	40.3	44.6	42.9	34.4	45.7	50.0	47.8	39.6	0	8	8

State	Alignment Scores of State Policies with IOM Standards								Scope of State Policies		
	Overall Score[a] (out of 100)				Nutrient Standards Only Score[b] (out of 100)				No. of IOM Standards Fully Met (out of 13)	No. of IOM Standards Partially Met (out of 13)	Total Scope
	All School Levels	E	M	H	All School Levels	E	M	H			
New York[e]	3.4	3.6	3.6	3.1	4.3	4 3	4.3	4.2	0	1	1
North Carolina	22.2	39.3	16.1	12.5	27.1	45.7	19.6	16.7	0	6	6
North Dakota[c]											
Ohio	23.3	25.0	25.0	20.3	24 3	26.1	26.1	20.8	0	5	5
Oklahoma[e]	4.5	7.1	7.1	0	5.7	8.7	8.7	0	0	1	1
Oregon	41.5	44.6	44.6	35.9	47.1	50.0	50.0	41.7	1	6	7
Pennsylvania[d]	0	0	0	0	0	0	0	0	0	0	0
Rhode Island	40.3	41.1	41.1	39.1	47.9	47.8	47.8	47.9	1	5	6
South Carolina	11.4	35.7	0	0	14 3	43.5	0	0	0	5	5
South Dakota[c]											
Tennessee	30.7	48.2	48 2	0	35.7	54.3	54 3	0	0	10	10
Texas	29.5	35.7	28.6	25.0	37.1	43.5	34.8	33.3	1	5	6
Utah[d]	0	0	0	0	0	0	0	0	0	0	0
Vermont[d]	0	0	0	0	0	0	0	0	0	0	0
Virginia[f]	0	0	0	0	0	0	0	0	0	0	0
Washington	33.0	33.9	33.9	31.3	38.6	39.1	39.1	37.5	0	4	4
West Virginia	60.2	62.5	62 5	56.3	62.1	65.2	65 2	56.3	6	6	12
Wisconsin[c]											
Wyoming[c]											
STATE MEDIAN	25.6	32.1	25.0	17.2	28.6	37.0	28 3	16.7			
Range	0–70.5	0–71.4	0–71.4	0–68.8	0–76.4	0–80.4	0–76.1	0–77.1			

E = elementary school, M = middle school, H = high school.

[a] Overall alignment score is based on the sum of all variables for each applicable grade level, divided by 176 points (the maximum possible score), multiplied by 100 for ease of interpretation. Score for each grade level is based on the sum of applicable variables for each grade level, divided by the maximum possible score for each grade level (E = 56, M = 56, H = 64), multiplied by 100 for ease of interpretation.

[b] Nutrient standards only alignment score is based on the sum of 24 variables for each applicable grade level, divided by 140 points (the maximum possible score), multiplied by 100 for ease of interpretation. Score for each grade level is based on the sum of applicable variables for each grade level, divided by the maximum possible score for each grade level (E = 46, M = 46, H = 48), multiplied by 100 for ease of interpretation.

[c] No state policy for competitive foods.

[d] Michigan, Pennsylvania, Utah, and Vermont have state policies for competitive foods, but these policies are voluntary or only recommended for school districts to implement. Connecticut's competitive beverage standards are required, but competitive food standards are voluntary.

[e] State policy for competitive foods only has exemptions for foods of minimal nutritional value (FMNV). Maine has additional restrictions on competitive foods, but these are not clearly defined.

[f] Massachusetts and Virginia enacted legislation requiring their state education/health agencies to develop state nutrition standards for competitive foods in schools. These standards were not available at the time of this analysis. Massachusetts' policy requires several elements to be included in the state standards. Two of these elements relate to nutrition standards—the availability of water at no cost and the availability of fruits and vegetables. These elements were coded.

A Closer Look at Each Institute of Medicine Standard

The IOM Standards that were most commonly met in state policies, either fully or partially (across all grade levels combined), were as follows (see Figure 4):

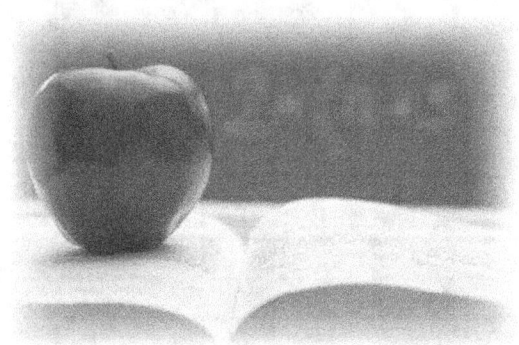

- **Standard 7:** Tier 1 Foods (34 states).

- **Standard 1:** Dietary Fat (25 states).

- **Standard 2:** Total Sugars (25 states).

- **Standard 9:** Sport Drinks (24 states).

- **Standard 13:** Fund-raising (21 states).

- **Standard 3:** Calories (21 states).

The IOM Standards that were least commonly met in state policies, either fully or partially, were as follows (see Figure 4):

- **Standard 10:** Reward or Discipline (3 states).

- **Standard 11:** Marketing (3 states).

- **Standard 5:** Nonnutritive Sweeteners (10 states).

- **Standard 6:** Caffeine (10 states).

- **Standard 4:** Sodium (10 states).

- **Standard 12:** After School (10 states).

- **Standard 8:** Water (13 states).

Only four of the IOM Standards were fully met by more than one state policy:

- **Standard 9:** Sports Drinks (7 states).

- **Standard 1:** Dietary Fat (4 states).

- **Standard 2:** Total Sugars (3 states).

- **Standard 3:** Calories (2 states).

Figure 4. Number of States that Fully Met, Partially Met, or Did Not Meet Each Institute of Medicine Standard

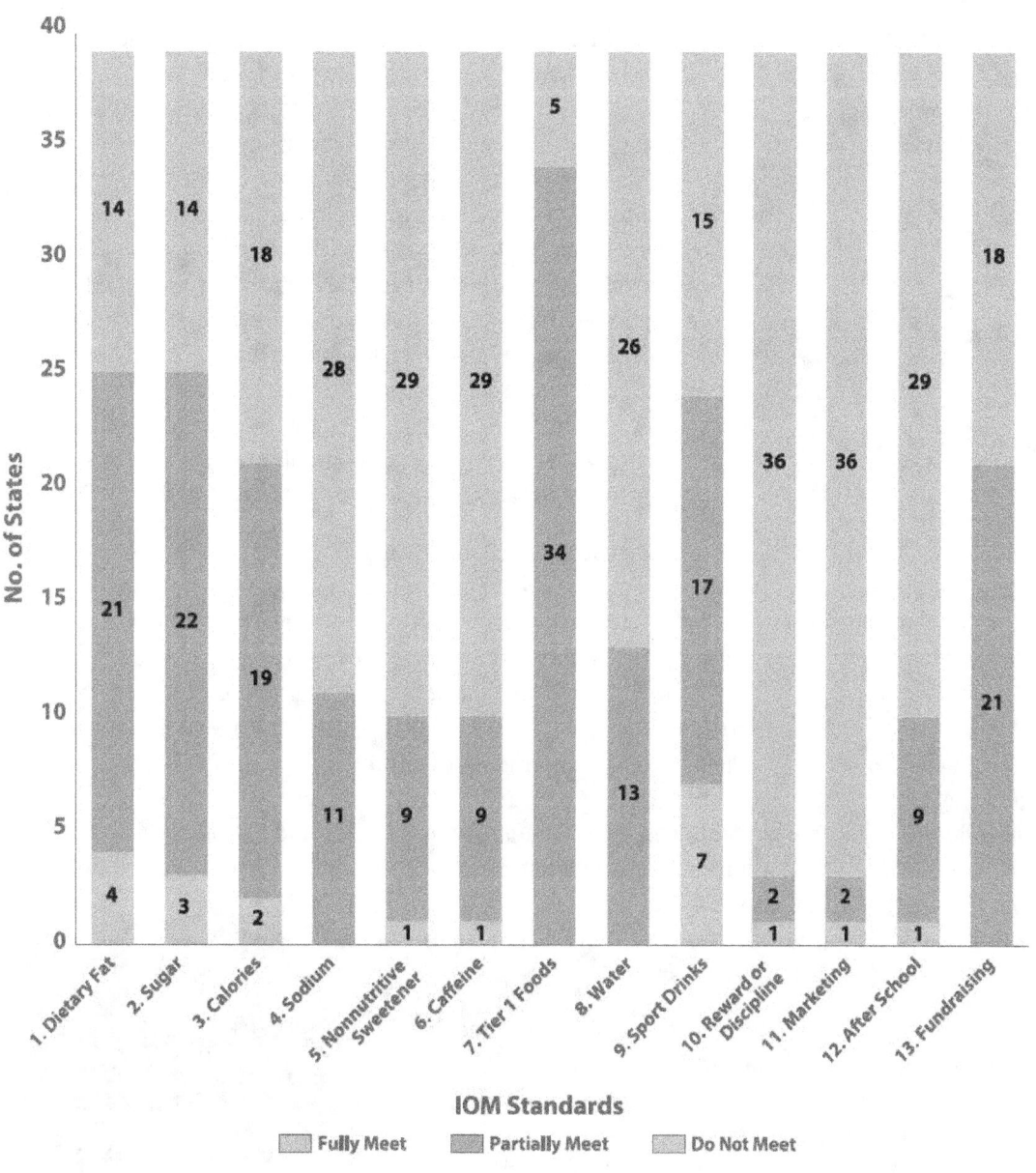

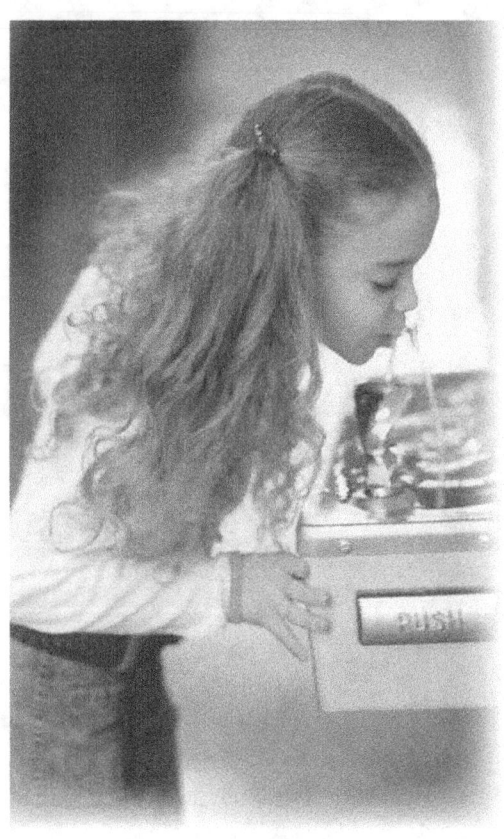

Discussion

Many schools and school districts have improved the nutritional quality of competitive foods and beverages during the past decade. However, studies have found room for improvement.[12-14] Competitive foods have the potential to undermine the effect of federally reimbursable school meal programs and may contribute to the increasing problem of childhood obesity because these foods tend to be calorie-dense.[15] In addition, school officials and others are concerned that offering healthier options for competitive foods and beverages, or not selling any competitive foods, will result in a loss of revenue from the sale of these foods and beverages. Although some schools report an initial decrease in revenue after implementing stronger nutrition standards, a growing body of evidence suggests that schools can have strong nutrition standards and maintain financial stability.[9,16,17]

Given the amount of time that children spend in school, the school environment can greatly influence students' attitudes, preferences, and behaviors towards healthy eating. Studies have reported that when school-aged children eat and drink foods and beverages high in fat, salt, and sugar, it can displace their consumption of healthier foods (e.g., fruits, vegetables) and beverages (e.g., low-fat or nonfat milk).[5,6] Schools play a critical role by providing opportunities for young people to be exposed to a variety of healthy foods and beverages, helping students develop good eating habits, and teaching them about the importance of healthy eating. The development of good eating habits at an early age should be encouraged because it can have a beneficial effect on children's school performance and helps them maintain a healthy lifestyle as adults.[18,19]

However, students receive mixed messages when foods and beverages sold in their schools do not align with the nutrition education they receive, or when unhealthy foods are marketed to them in their schools.

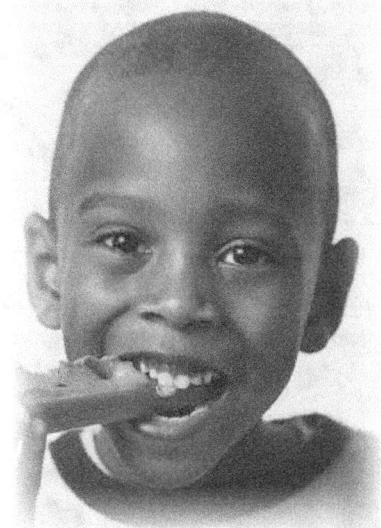

This analysis included state policies for competitive foods in schools, required or voluntary. Policies for Michigan, Pennsylvania, Utah, and Vermont had alignment scores in the 1st quartile, indicating lowest alignment with IOM Standards because they were voluntary. States such as Delaware, Georgia, Maine, Maryland, New York, and Oklahoma also had policies with lower alignment scores because their policies only restricted FMNV beyond the current federal regulations for some grade levels and did not have required nutrition standards for other competitive foods and beverages.

In Massachusetts and Virginia, state officials enacted policies for competitive foods in schools before October 1, 2010, but these standards were still under development at the time of this analysis. As a result, the alignment scores for these policies are in the 1st quartile (lowest alignment).

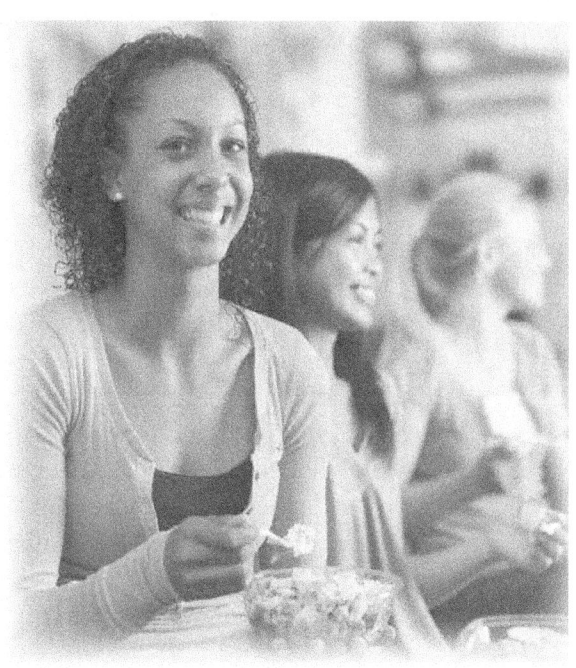

In addition to policy requirements, financial incentives are a promising way to increase implementation of competitive food standards that may be voluntary, as with Pennsylvania and Connecticut state policies. Pennsylvania enacted legislation in 2007 that provides a supplemental reimbursement for each breakfast and lunch served as part of the School Breakfast Program and the National School Lunch Program, to schools that adopt, implement, or exceed the Pennsylvania Department of Education's voluntary nutrition guidelines for foods and beverages available on campus. Connecticut reimburses schools with an additional 10 cents per lunch if they meet the state's voluntary Healthy Food Certification program. Connecticut's state policy only requires school districts to meet beverage standards.

The results of this analysis show that state policies for competitive foods and beverages in schools vary in their alignment with IOM Standards and the scope of their standards. Overall, the majority of state policies have alignment scores that are in the 1st and 2nd quartiles (i.e., below the 50th percentile). Although some state policies incorporate elements of the IOM Standards for competitive foods and beverages, no state fully met half (7 or more) of the 13 IOM Standards for all school levels. Overall, state policies for middle and high schools were less aligned with IOM Standards compared with policies for elementary schools. This finding is mirrored at the local/district level.[13,14]

This analysis has several potential limitations. The study examines the language in codified laws and state board of education policies, memos, and resolutions, not the actual implementation or compliance with a policy or other actions at the district or school level to improve the quality of competitive foods in schools. Secondly, researchers relied on government Web sites to obtain codified laws and state board of education policy documents, some of which may not be completely up-to-date.

The IOM Standards released in 2007 were used as the gold standard for coding and analyzing state policies. Some states that enacted policies before 2007 might have been at a disadvantage compared with other states because the information on the recommended standards was not available at the time they adopted their policies. In addition, although state policies received separate alignment scores for each school level, they did not receive separate scores for different venues (e.g., vending machines, school stores, à la carte food items). Examining policy alignment by venue could provide states with additional and more specific information on how to improve their alignment with IOM Standards.

A further limitation is that all IOM Standards were not given equal weight. Standards were divided into variables depending on their complexity. For example, IOM Standard 7 was divided into 11 variables, whereas Standard 1 was only divided into 3 variables, allowing Standard 7 to add greater weight to the overall alignment score. Although the IOM did not rank the 13 standards in order of importance, Standard 7 was given more weight because it encompasses IOM Standards 1–6 and 9.

Implications for Practice

The Healthy, Hunger-Free Kids Act of 2010 authorizes the U.S. Department of Agriculture to develop federal standards for competitive foods in schools that align with the most up-to-date science. The results of this study can be used to aid the development of these new federal standards and to provide technical assistance to states. 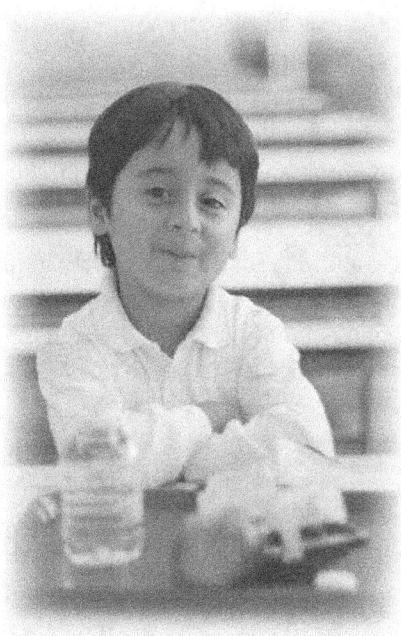 The federal government and states can use this information to identify differences across grade levels and competitive food and beverage standards that are less likely to be included in state policies, such as the standards on sodium and water.

All states can demonstrate leadership by developing state policies that align with IOM Standards for foods and beverages sold outside the school meals program.

References

1. Ogden CL, Carroll MD, Curtin LR, Lamb MM, Flegal KM. Prevalence of high body mass index in U.S. children and adolescents, 2007–2008. *JAMA* 2010;303(3):242–249.

2. Briefel RR, Crepinsek MK, Cabili C, Wilson A, Gleason PM. School food environments and practices affect dietetic behaviors of US public school children. *Journal of the American Dietetic Association* 2009;109(Suppl 1):S91–S107.

3. Fox MK, Dodd AH, Wilson A, Gleason PM. Association between school food environment and practices and body mass index of US public school children. *Journal of the American Dietetic Association* 2009;109(Suppl 2): S108–S117.

4. Fox MK, Gordon A, Nogales R, Wilson A. Availability and consumption of competitive foods in US public schools. *Journal of the American Dietetic Association* 2009;109:S57–S66.

5. Kubik MY, Lytle LA, Hannan PJ, Perry CL, Story M. The association of the school food environment with dietary behaviors of young adolescents. *American Journal of Public Health* 2003;93(7):1168–1173.

6. Storey ML, Forshee RA, Anderson PA. Associations of adequate intake of calcium with diet, beverage consumption, and demographic characteristics among children and adolescents. *Journal of the American College of Nutrition* 2004;23(1):18–33.

7. National School Lunch Program. *Federal Register*. 2006. To be codified at 7 CFR §210.

8. School Breakfast Program. *Federal Register*. 2006. To be codified at 7 CFR §220.

9. Government Accountability Office. School Meal Programs: Competitive Foods Are Widely Available and Generate Substantial Revenues for Schools. Washington, DC: Government Accountability Office;2005. GAO Publication no. GAO-05-563.

10. Chriqui JF, Schneider L, Chaloupka FJ, Pugach O. *Local wellness policies: assessing school district strategies for improving children's health. School years 2006–07 and 2007–08*. Chicago, IL: University of Illinois at Chicago; 2009. Available at http://www.bridgingthegapresearch.org/research/district_wellness_policies.

11. Institute of Medicine. Nutrition Standards for Foods in Schools: Leading the Way Toward Healthier Youth. Washington, DC: National Academies Press; 2007.

12. O'Toole TP, Anderson S, Miller C, Guthrie J. Nutrition services and foods and beverages available at school: results from the school health policies and programs study 2006. *Journal of School Health* 2007;77(8):500–521.

13. Finkelstein DM, Hill EL, Whitaker RC. School food environments and policies in US public schools. *Pediatrics* 2008;122(1):e251–e259.

14. Chriqui JF, Schneider L, Chaloupka FJ, et al. *School district wellness policies: evaluating progress and potential for improving children's health three years after the federal mandate. School years 2006–07, 2007–08, and 2008–09*. Vol. 2. Chicago: University of Illinois at Chicago; 2010. Available at http://www.bridgingthegapresearch.org/research/district_wellness_policies.

15. Kubik MA, Lytle LA, Story M. School-wide food practices are associated with body mass index in middle school students. *Archives of Pediatrics and Adolescent Medicine* 2005;159:1111–1114.

16. Centers for Disease Control and Prevention. *Implementing Strong Nutrition Standards for Schools: Financial Implications*. Atlanta: U.S. Department of Health and Human Services; 2011. Available at http://www.cdc.gov/healthyyouth/nutrition/pdf/financial_implications.pdf.

17. Wharton CM, Long M, Schwartz MB. Changing nutrition standards in schools: the emerging impact on school revenue. *Journal of School Health* 2008;78:245–251.

18. Florence MD, Asbridge M, Veugelers PJ. Diet quality and academic performance. *Journal of School Health* 2008;78:209–215.

19. Story M, Nanney MS, Schwartz MB. Schools and obesity prevention: creating school environments and policies to promote healthy eating and physical activity. *Milbank Quarterly* 2009;87(1):71–100.

Appendix A.
Institute of Medicine (IOM) Standards and Related Variables

IOM Standards	Variables		E[a] (max score)	M[a] (max score)	H[a] (max score)
Standard 1 Snacks, foods, and beverages meet criteria for dietary fat per portion packaged.	1.	Snacks, foods, and beverages provide ≤35% total calories from fat per portion as packaged.[b]	2	2	2
	2.	Snacks, foods, and beverages provide <10% total calories from saturated fat per portion as packaged.[b]	2	2	2
	3.	Snacks, foods, and beverages contain zero trans fat per portion as packaged.[b]	2	2	2
Standard 2 Snacks, foods, and beverages provide ≤35% calories from total sugars per portion as packaged.	4.	Snacks, foods, and beverages provide ≤35% calories from total sugars per portion as packaged.[b]	2	2	2
Standard 3 Snack items are ≤200 calories per portion as packaged and à la carte entrée items do not exceed calorie limits on comparable NSLP[c] items.	5.	Snack items contain ≤200 calories per portion as packaged.[b]	2	2	2
	6.	À la carte entrée items do not exceed calorie limits on comparable NSLP items.[b]	2	2	2
Standard 4 Snack items meet a sodium content limit of ≤200 mg per portion as packaged or ≤480 mg per entrée portion as served for à la carte.	7.	Snack items meet a sodium content limit of ≤200 mg per portion as packaged.[b]	2	2	2
	8.	À la carte entrée items contain ≤480 mg sodium per entrée portion as served.[b]	2	2	2
Standard 5 Beverages containing nonnutritive sweeteners are only allowed in high schools after the end of the school day.	9.	Beverages containing nonnutritive sweeteners are only allowed in high schools after the end of the school day.[b]	*	*	2
Standard 6 Foods and beverages are caffeine-free, with the exception of trace amounts of naturally occurring caffeine-related substances.	10.	Foods and beverages are caffeine-free.[b]	2	2	2

IOM Standards	Variables	E[a] (max score)	M[a] (max score)	H[a] (max score)
Standard 7 Foods and beverages offered during the school day are limited to Tier 1[d] foods and beverages.	11. Fruits and vegetables.[b]	2	2	2
	12. Whole grains.[b]	2	2	2
	13. Nonfat or low-fat dairy products.[b]	2	2	2
	14. 100% fruit and vegetable juices (E = 4 oz max; M, H = 8 oz max).[b]	2	2	2
	15. Nonfat or low-fat milk (E, M, H = 8 oz max).[b]	2	2	2
	16. Flavored milk, max 22g total sugars/8 oz (E, M, H = 8 oz max).[b]	2	2	2
	17. Prohibits regular (sugar-sweetened) soda.[b]	2	2	2
	18. Prohibits other beverages (other than soda and sport drinks) that contain added caloric sweetener.[b]	2	2	2
	19. Prohibits FMNV[e] all day throughout school campus.[b]	2	2	2
	20. Allows Tier 1 foods only in addition to meeting all other IOM nutrient standards.[b]	2	2	2
	21. Allows Tier 1 beverages only in addition to meeting all other IOM nutrient standards.[b]	2	2	2
Standard 8 Plain, potable water is available throughout the school day at no cost to students.	22. Requires the availability of water (bottled, tap, or fountain) at no cost throughout the school day.[b]	2	2	2
	23. Prohibits carbonated, fortified, and flavored waters.[b]	2	2	2
Standard 9 Sports drinks are not available in the school setting.	24. Prohibits sports drinks in the school setting.[b]	2	2	2
Standard 10 Foods and beverages are not used as rewards or discipline for academic performance or behavior.	25. Prohibits foods and beverages from being used as rewards.	2	2	2
	26. Prohibits foods and beverages from being used as discipline.	*	*	2
Standard 11 Minimizes marketing of Tier 2[f] foods and beverages in high school setting.	27. Minimizes marketing by locating Tier 2 foods and beverages in low student traffic areas in high school.	*	*	2
	28. Minimizes marketing by ensuring exterior of vending machines do not depict commercial products or logos or suggest that consumption of vended items conveys a health or social benefit in high school.	2	2	*
Standard 12 Tier 1 snack items are allowed after school for student activities for elementary and middle schools. Tier 1 and 2 snacks are allowed after school in high school.	29. Allows Tier 1 snacks for after school for student activities in elementary and middle schools.	2	2	*
	30. Allows Tier 1 and 2 snacks after school in high school.	*	*	2

IOM Standards	Variables	E[a] (max score)	M[a] (max score)	H[a] (max score)
Standard 13 For on-campus fund-raising activities during the school day, Tier 1 foods and beverages are allowed for elementary, middle, and high schools. Tier 2 foods and beverages are allowed for high schools after school. For evening and community activities that include adults, Tier 1 and 2 foods and beverages are encouraged.	31. Allows sale of Tier 1 foods and beverages during on-campus fund-raising activities.	2	2	2
	32. Allows sale of Tier 2 foods and beverages on campus after school in high school.	*	*	2
	33. Encourages sale of Tier 1 and 2 foods and beverages during evening and community events that include adults.	2	2	2
Totals				
Number of variables by school level.	N = 33	28	28	32
	N = 24[b]	23[b]	23[b]	24[b]
Total maximum score by school level.		56	56	64
		46[b]	46[b]	48[b]
Total maximum score for all variables and all school levels combined.			176	
			140[b]	

* Not applicable.

[a] E = elementary school; M = middle school; H = high school.

[b] Indicates variables included in the nutrient standards only analysis and related maximum scores for each school level.

[c] National School Lunch Program.

[d] Tier 1 foods, which are for all students, are fruits, vegetables, whole grains, and related combination products and nonfat and low-fat dairy products that are limited to ≤200 calories per portion as packaged and ≤35% of total calories from fat, <10% of total calories from saturated fats, zero trans fat (≤0.5 g per serving), ≤35% of calories from total sugars, and ≤200 mg sodium. À la carte entrée items meet the same fat and sugar limits. Tier 1 beverages are water without flavoring, additives, or carbonation; low-fat and nonfat milk in 8-oz portions, including lactose-free and soy beverages and flavored milk with no more than 22 g of total sugars per 8-oz portion; 100% fruit juice in 4-oz portions as packaged for elementary/middle school and 8-oz portions for high school; and caffeine-free, with the exception of trace amounts of naturally occurring caffeine substances.

[e] Foods of minimal nutritional value.

[f] Tier 2 foods and beverages are any foods or beverages for high school students after school. Tier 2 snack foods are those that do not exceed 200 calories per portion as packaged and ≤35% of total calories from fat, <10% of total calories from saturated fats, zero trans fat (≤0.5 g per serving), ≤35% calories from total sugars, and a sodium content of ≤200 mg per portion as packaged. Tier 2 beverages are noncaffeinated, nonfortified beverages with <5 calories per portion as packaged, with or without nonnutritive sweeteners, carbonation, or flavoring.

Appendix B.
Citations of State Policies Analyzed

State	Policy Citations
Alabama	Alabama Administrative Code 290-080-030-.03
	Resolution on the Recommendations of the Committee to Review the State of Health of America's Youth with Particular Emphasis on Alabama's Youth—July 12, 2005 adopted
	Resolution Adopting Beverage Standards for Vending Sales in Alabama Public Schools—June 14, 2007 adopted
	State Board of Education Policy Memo, Nov 1 2001, Log # FY02-3005 (food)
Alaska	No policy
Arizona	Arizona Revised Statutes § 15-242
Arkansas	Arkansas Code Annotated § 20-7-135
California	California Education Code §§ 49430-49436
	California Code of Regulations Title 5 §§ 15500, 15501, 15575-15578
Colorado	Colorado Revised Statutes § 22-32-134.5
	Colorado Revised Statutes § 22-32-136
Connecticut	Connecticut General Statutes Chapter 169 §§10-215e and 10-215f
	Connecticut General Statutes Chapter 170 §10-221q
Delaware	Delaware Administrative Code Title 14 800 §852
Florida	Florida Administrative Code 6A-7.0411
Georgia	Georgia Rules and Regulations 160-5-6-.01
Hawaii	Hawaii State Board of Education Policy #1110-6
	Hawaii State Board of Education Policy #6810
	State of Hawaii Wellness Guidelines
Idaho	No policy
Illinois	Illinois Administrative Code Title 23 §305.15
Indiana	Indiana Code §20-26-9-19
Iowa	Iowa Administrative Code 281-58.10
Kansas	Kansas Statutes §72-5128
	Kansas Education Regulation 91-26-1
	Kansas State Board of Education— May 10 2010 approved minutes
Kentucky	Kentucky Administrative Regulations Title 702 §6.090
	Kentucky Revised Statutes §158.854
Louisiana	Louisiana Administrative Code Title 28 Chapter XLIX §741
	Louisiana Revised Statute §17:197.1
Maine	Maine Code of Rules 05-071-51
	Maine Revised Statutes Title 20-A 6662
Maryland	Maryland Education Code Annotated § 7-423
	Maryland State Department of Education, Management and Operations Memo MOM012
Massachusetts	Massachusetts General Laws Chapter 111, §222
Michigan	Michigan State Board of Education Minutes Oct 2010

State	Policy Citations
Minnesota	No policy
Mississippi	Mississippi Code Annotated § 37-13-134 and 137 Mississippi State Board of Education Policy #2002 (Competitive Food), #4003 (Beverage Regulations), and #4004 (Snack Regulations)
Missouri	No policy
Montana	No policy
Nebraska	No policy
Nevada	Nevada State Board of Education Approved Minutes June 17–18, 2005 Nevada State Department of Education Statewide Wellness Policy
New Hampshire	No policy
New Jersey	New Jersey Administrative Code Title 2, 36-1.7 and 36-1.11
New Mexico	New Mexico Administrative Code §6.12.5 New Mexico Statutes Annotated §22-13-13.1
New York	New York Education Code §915
North Carolina	North Carolina Administrative Code Title 16 6H.0104 North Carolina General Statutes §115C-264.2
North Dakota	No policy
Ohio	Ohio Revised Code §§3313.814, 816, 817 Ohio Administrative Code §3301-91-09
Oklahoma	Oklahoma Statutes Annotated §70-5-147 Oklahoma Administrative Code §210:10-3-111
Oregon	Oregon Revised Statutes Chapter 336 §423 Oregon Administrative Rules 581-051-0100
Pennsylvania	Pennsylvania Public School Code §1337.1
Rhode Island	Rhode Island General Laws §§16-21-7 and 16-21-29
South Carolina	South Carolina Code of Laws §§59-10-310 and 59-10-330 South Carolina Code of Regulations §43-168
South Dakota	No policy
Tennessee	Tennessee Code Annotated §49-6-2307 Tennessee Rules and Regulations 0520-1-6.04
Texas	Texas Administrative Code Title 4 §§26.1-26.9
Utah	Utah Administrative Code 277-719
Vermont	Vermont Act 203 Section 16
Virginia	Virginia Administrative Code Title 8 §20-290-10
Washington	Washington Revised Code §28A.210.365
West Virginia	West Virginia Code of State Rules §§126-86-1 to 126-86-16 West Virginia Code §18-2-6a West Virginia State Board of Education Policy 4321.1
Wisconsin	No policy
Wyoming	No policy

Nutrition Facts

Serving Size 2 pieces (30g)

Total Fat

Sodium

Total Carb. 2g

Sugars 0g

Sugar Alco

Protein

U.S Department of Health and Human Services

Centers for Disease Control and Prevention

2012

CS225610-B

www.ingramcontent.com/pod-product-compliance
Lightning Source LLC
Chambersburg PA
CBHW081812170526
45167CB00008B/3405